I0440078

21 Super Healthy Herbs

Magic herbs for herbs that heal and herbs in the kitchen

Ellen Vincent

© 2013 by *Ellen Vincent*

All rights reserved.

All Rights Reserved. No part of this publication may be reproduced in any form or by any means, including scanning, photocopying, or otherwise without prior written permission of the copyright holder.

Disclaimer and Terms of Use: The Author and Publisher has strived to be as accurate and complete as possible in the creation of this book, notwithstanding the fact that she does not warrant or represent at any time that the contents within are accurate due to the rapidly changing nature of the Internet and science. While all attempts have been made to verify information provided in this publication, the Author and Publisher assumes no responsibility for errors, omissions, or contrary interpretation of the subject matter herein. Any perceived slights of specific persons, peoples, or organizations are unintentional. In practical advice books, like anything else in life, there are no guarantees of results produced. Readers are cautioned to rely on their own judgment about their individual circumstances and to act accordingly and if necessary seek professional help and advice.

First Printing, 2010

ISBN -13:978-1490351070

ISBN -10:1490351078

Printed in the United States of America

21 Super Healthy Herbs

Magic herbs for herbs that heal and herbs in the kitchen

Table of Contents

Introduction

Herbs are a valuable health resource that shouldn't be ignored. Herbs have been used in medicine for thousands of years and are still being used today. Most of the drugs that are used by doctors to treat us are of plant origin. Scientists continually search far off places such as the upper reaches of the Amazon for new plants that might provide future chemical compounds for use in the treatment of diseases such as cancer.

Even universally used medicines, such as the pain killer Aspirin have their origin in plant material. Leaves provided by the humble willow tree gave rise to Aspirin. Now there is renewed interest in even those basic herbs that we use in cooking to flavor our food. The Mediterranean diet is one that has been proved to be of great benefit in preventing illnesses such as heart disease and cancer and fresh herbs are an essential part of this regimen. Doctors in the UK often recommend adding herbs such as Turmeric to your diet because of their anti cancer properties. Use herbs as a flavor enhancer instead of salt and you will be helping yourself even more. The World Health Organization pronounced that salt is one of the biggest killers in the world today.

Take a look at these 21 super herbs and add them to your meals so that you too can have the health benefits of herb power. Herbs also make your food taste better too. Herbs can be your answer to fantastic tasting food without salt. Each herb has a full color image and a description of the health benefits that you find on using them.

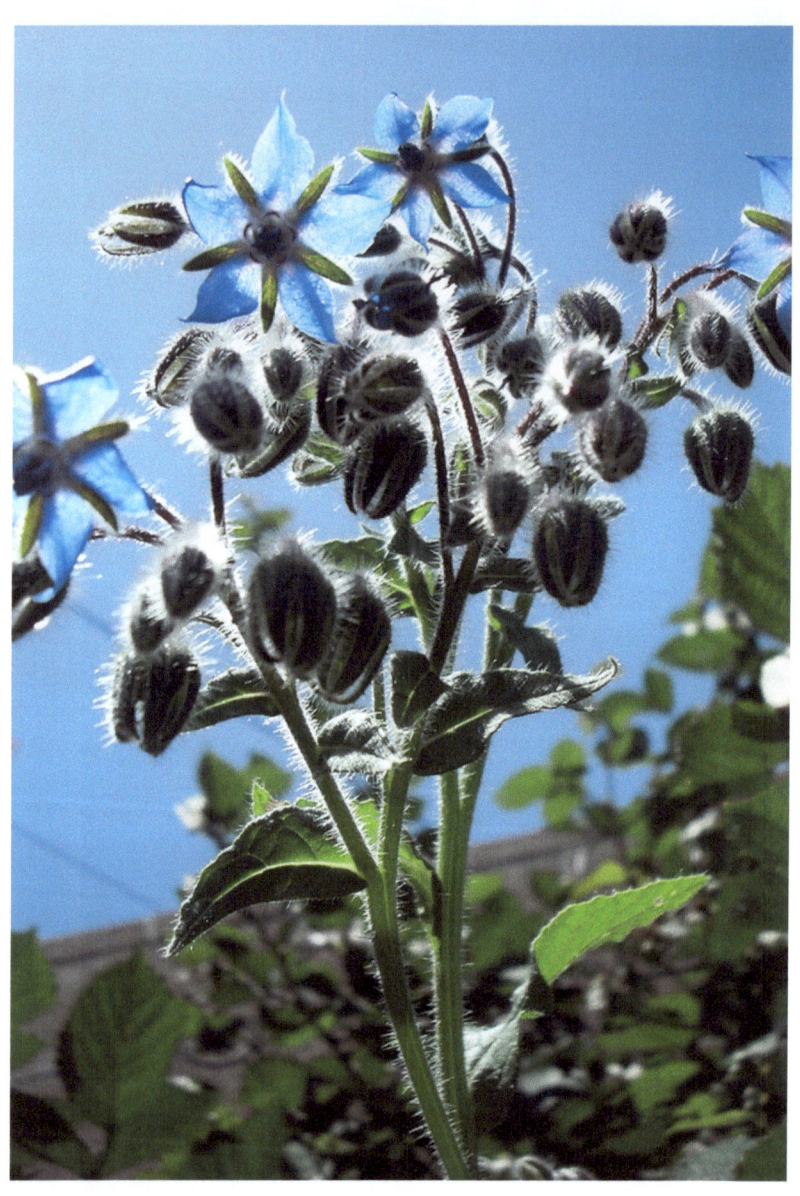

Borage

Description

Borage is an annual herb that has hollow stems covered in hair like bristles. The plant can be up to 30 inches in height. The leaves are large and oval in shape with a covering of furry hairs. It has star shaped blue flowers. It will grow in most places but is very abundant in Anatolia and Eastern Europe.

Health benefits

Borage contains Gamma Linolenic acid which is important in the health of the joints, skin and immune system. The fresh herb contains large amounts of Vitamin C which is an important antioxidant which boosts the immune system helping it deal with wounds and virus pathogens such as those involved in colds and influenza. It also has a lot of Vitamin A and Carotenes which are also powerful antioxidants. These can help in reducing the effects of ageing. It can help with vision and skin health. Vitamin A is also a substance that has anti cancer properties. . Borage contains a lot of minerals and is especially high in iron, calcium, manganese and potassium. It has a high vitamin B content which means that it is good for lowering Cholesterol levels and promoting metabolism in the body.

How to use

The young Borage leaves are tender and can be used in salads where it provides a cucumber like flavor. The older leaves which are tougher and bitterer tasting can be used as vegetable greens in cooking and is rather similar to spinach. The leaves can be added to sausage meat and poultry stuffing. It can be added to pizza toppings. You can also steep the leaves in hot water to make a refreshing tea.

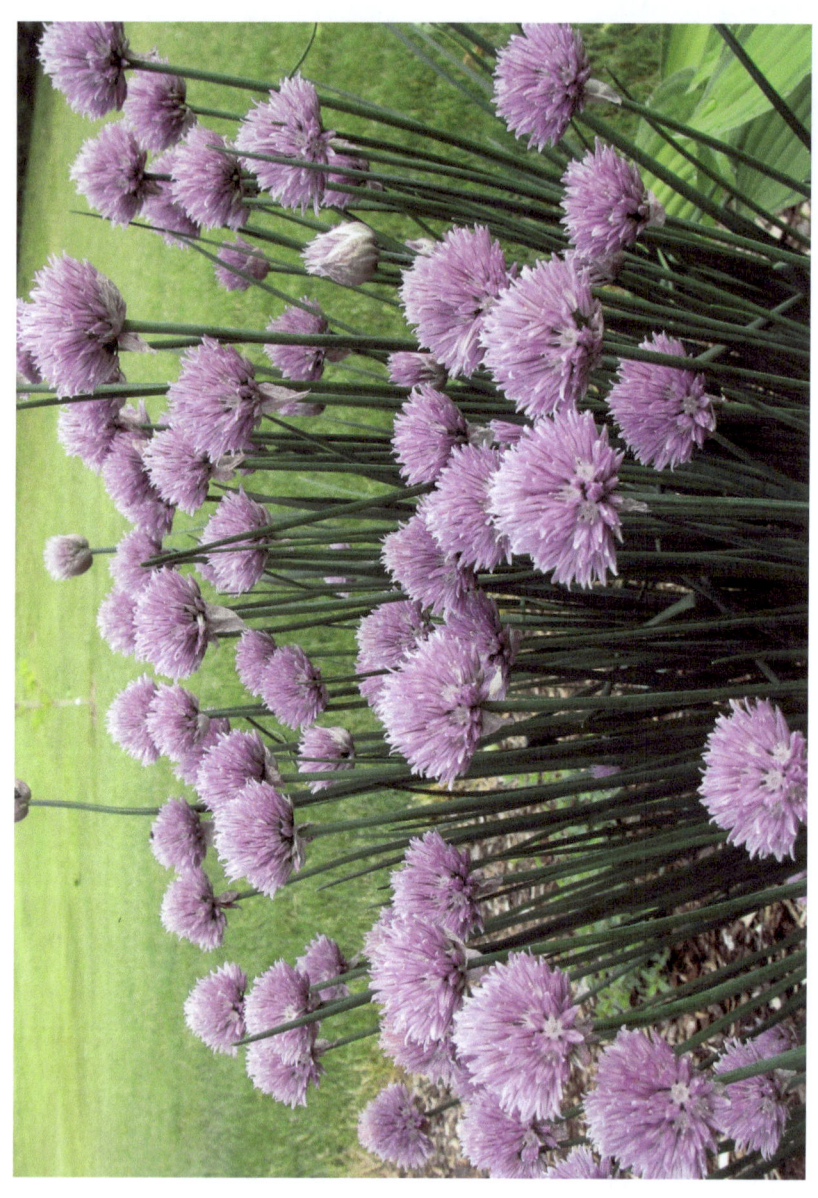

Chives

Description

Chives have a sweet and mild onion flavor. The leaves are hollow like spring onions but they aren't as big in diameter and may a look a little like grass. Unlike onions only the leaves are used. They are available to use all year round.

Health benefits

Chives contain a number of interesting substances including a lot of fiber. When the leaves are cut or crushed they release a substance called allicin which can help to reduce cholesterol levels in the body. Allicin also has antimicrobial properties as well as the ability to reduce blood pressure and reduce blood clotting within blood vessels. This means that it can help to prevent cardiovascular disease and strokes. Vitamins A, K, B complex and C are found in chives which mean that it is good for helping with ageing and even Alzheimer's. Chives contain a lot of folic acid which is good at protecting the health of unborn babies.

How to use

Chives are widely used in Mediterranean and French food. Their flavor isn't overpowering and can add a vibrant green color to a range of dishes. Leaves should be cut and served at the last minute to reduce the loss of the chive flavor. They work well with tomato salad and can easily be added to sandwiches, sauces and soups. Chives can be mixed with cream cheese and also as a garnish on cold dishes. You can also add them to such foods as pizza, omelets, quiche, muffins, scones and savory biscuits.

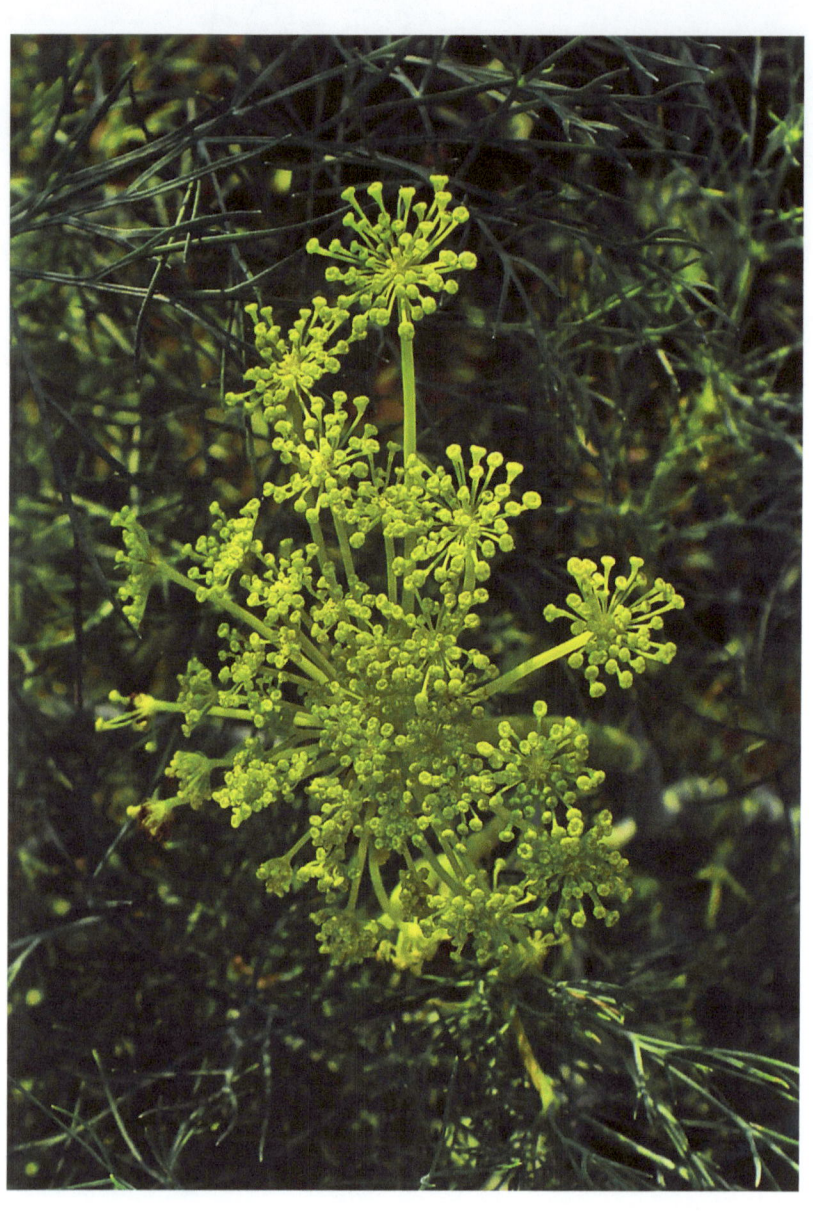

Dill Weed

Description

Dill Weed has feathery dark green leaves that look a little bit like ferns. These leaves smell lovely and are soft and sweet tasting. The leaves of Dill are used as a herb and seeds may be used as a spice.

Health benefits

Dill weed contains many helpful plant substances. It is high in Vitamin A and C. It contains antioxidants which are good at reducing ageing and fighting against diseases. This herb has few calories and is low in cholesterol. It contains a number of essential oils. Eugenol is one of these and this is thought to help to reduce blood sugar levels as well as having anesthetic and antiseptic properties. Dill contains a good range of minerals and is especially high in copper, manganese, calcium and iron. Dill leaves can help digestion and can help reduce flatulence as well.

How to use

Dill weed should be added to recipes quite near to serving because it lose its flavor and aromatic aroma. Dill has been used in recipes in the Mediterranean region for centuries. It is especially good with chicken, fish, meat and vegetable dishes. It can be used when making soups and sauces. Freshly chopped Dill is good with salads and it can also be sautéed with the ingredients or before adding to salads. Dill seeds and sprigs are often added to pickles for extra flavor.

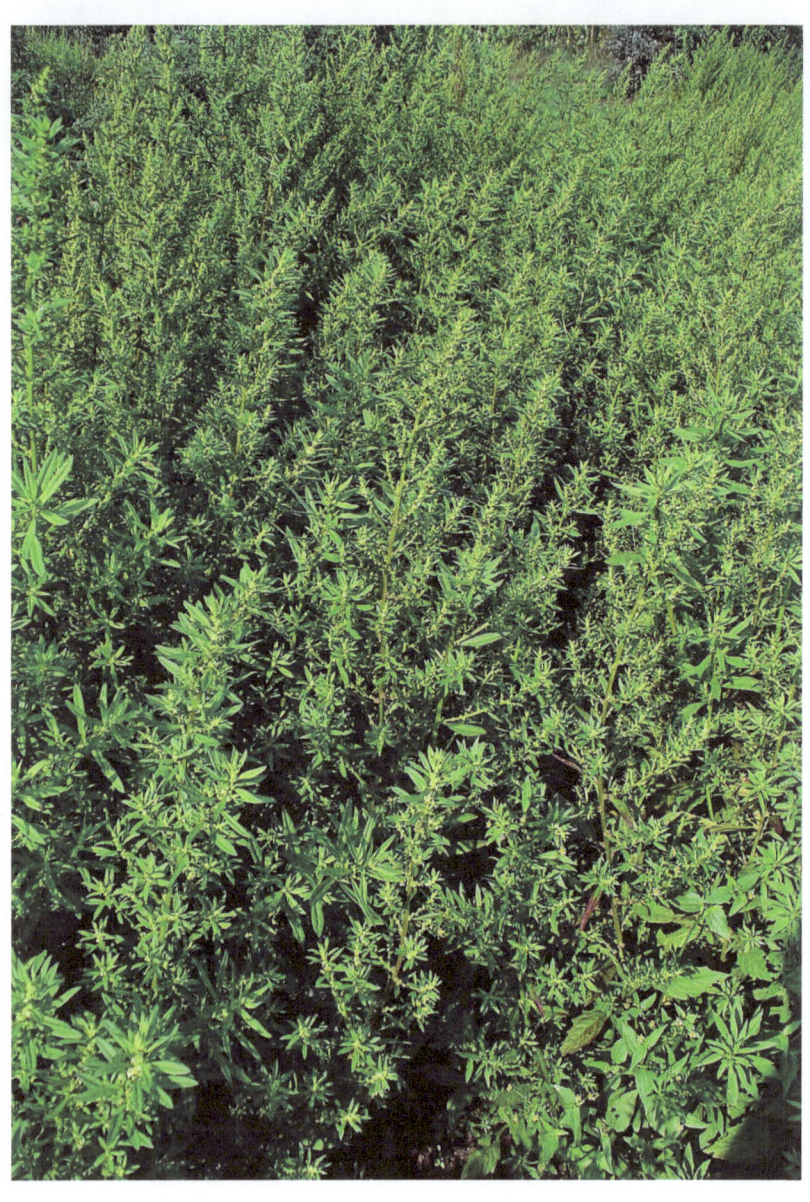

14

Epazote

Description

Epazote originated in Mexico and has been used by the people there for thousands of years. It still imparts a special taste to classic Mexican dishes. It has a hearty musk like flavor. It is an annual herb and grows to some 3 feet in height. The leaves are pointed and have serrated edges. It produces small yellow green flowers.

Health benefits

Typically Epazote has been used in recipes in order to deal with flatulence and digestive problems caused by the high fiber and protein diet provided by beans in the Mexican diet. Despite this, Epazote is also high in fiber as well as being low in calories as well.

It contains the compound Ascaridole which acts as a poison in the case of a number of parasitic worms found in the human intestine. Natives of the region take the herb in order to keep themselves free of such worms.

Although it is high in folic acid, which is good for developing babies in the womb, it can cause conditions such as uterine cramps and as a result pregnant women may be advised to avoid it in their diet.

This herb has a small amount of vitamins such as A and B complex, but is high in minerals such as calcium, Manganese and potassium.

How to use

The young shoots can be added to soups as a vegetable. The older leaves are best used to help with digestion in bean, corn and fish recipes. A herbal infusion of older leaves is often made and then added to recipes such as soups.

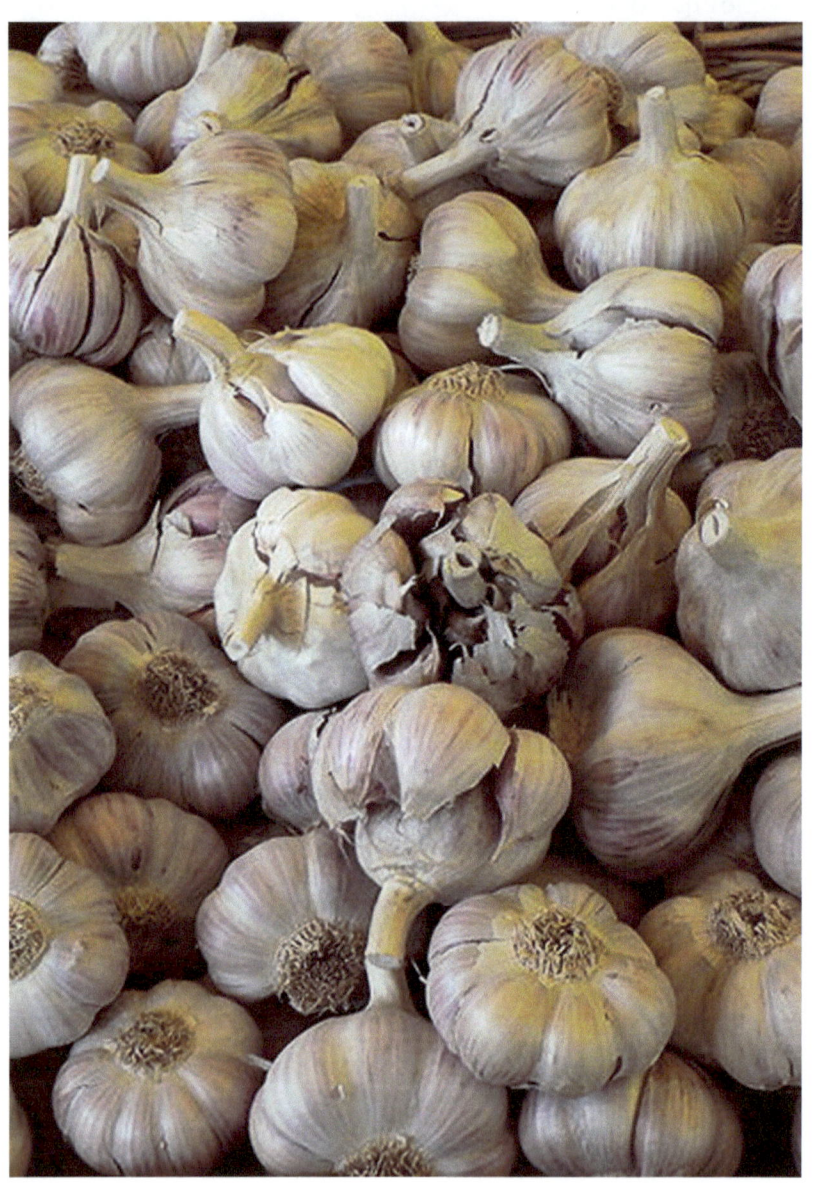

Garlic

Description

Garlic is a well known flavor enhancer used across the whole world. It is thought to have originated in central Asia but is now grown in most sub tropical areas. The root bulbils or cloves are typically used but the shoots are useful too.

Health benefits

Allicin is an important substance made within garlic cloves from thiosulphates when the cloves are cut or crushed. Allicin has been shown to reduce cholesterol production in the liver of people who eat it. Allicin also makes blood vessels more flexible which helps to reduce blood pressure. This means that it is helpful in the prevention of heart disease and strokes. Allicin together with other substances in garlic are also good at dealing with invading pathogens such as bacteria, viruses and fungi.

Garlic is rich in minerals. It has a lot of Selenium which is good for heart health. It also has a lot of manganese which is important for the production of red blood cells. Vitamins are also in good supply and garlic is rich in vitamin C and the antioxidants carotene and xanthin.

Garlic is often used in cold remedies and garlic oil can be used to treat fungal infections.

How to use

Use the leaves like you would green onion tops. The cloves are used as flavoring and seasoning of many dishes. Use to promote the flavor of seafood, meat and fish dishes. Rub onto toasted bread of Bruschettas and use in soups, sauces and stews.

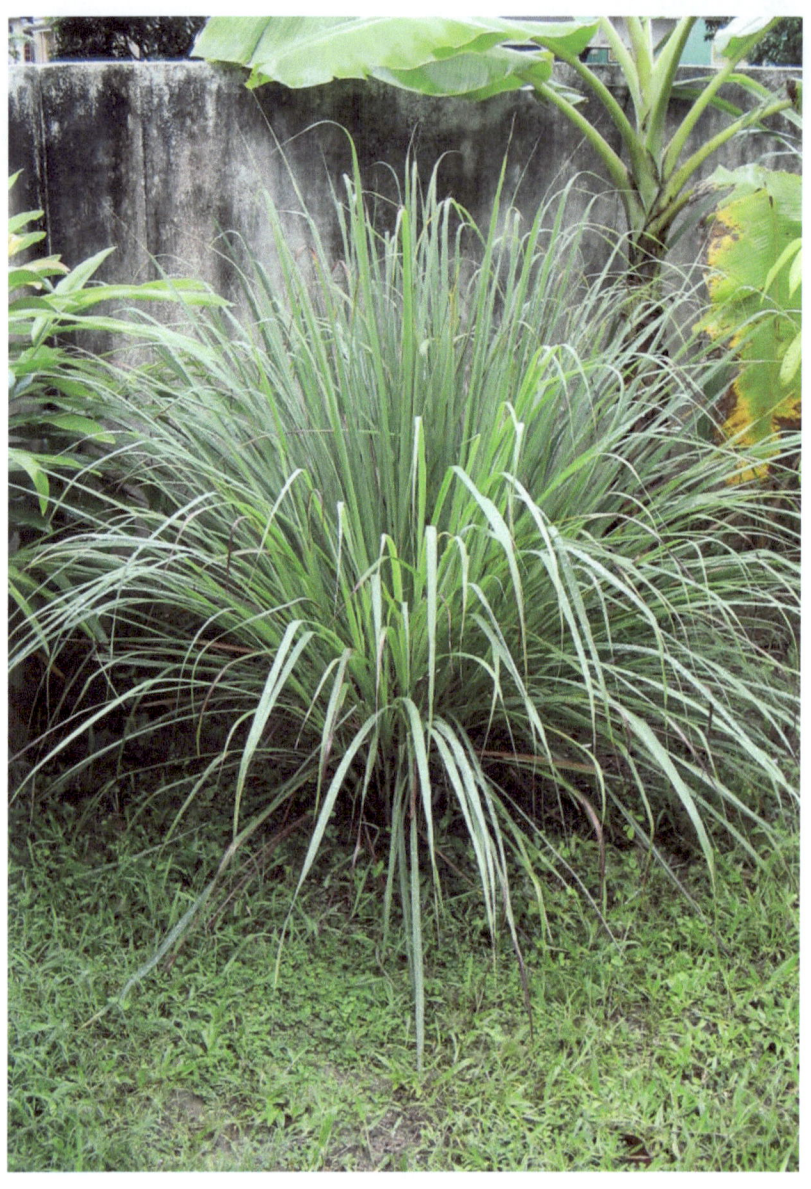

Lemongrass

Description

Lemongrass has a stimulating citrus aroma and gives a very individual flavor to food. The most used parts are the hairy stems and buds of the lemongrass plant. It is used to great effect in Southern Asian areas of the world. It has long leaves with sharp edges and grows to about 3 feet in height.

Health benefits

Lemongrass contains many substances that can have health benefits. The citral aroma compound can act as an antimicrobial agent. It contains essential oils such as myrocene and citronellol which can be used as an insecticide and to stop skin irritations. Folic acid is found in the stem and leaves and this has a beneficial effect on fetus growth in the womb by preventing birth defects.

It contains high levels of vitamins including B complexes, and smaller amounts of antioxidants such as vitamins C and A.

Lemongrass is rich in minerals like potassium, zinc, calcium and iron.

How to use

Lemongrass is used a lot in Asian cooking and its gentle flavor goes well with fish, seafood, meat and poultry. Its lemon flavor is released when the grass is cut or crushed. The tough stems can be removed before eating.

It is used a lot in soups, curries, sauces and stir fries in Thailand and surrounding countries.

You can make a refreshing tea by steeping the Lemongrass leaves in boiling water. It can also be used as a flavor when pickling.

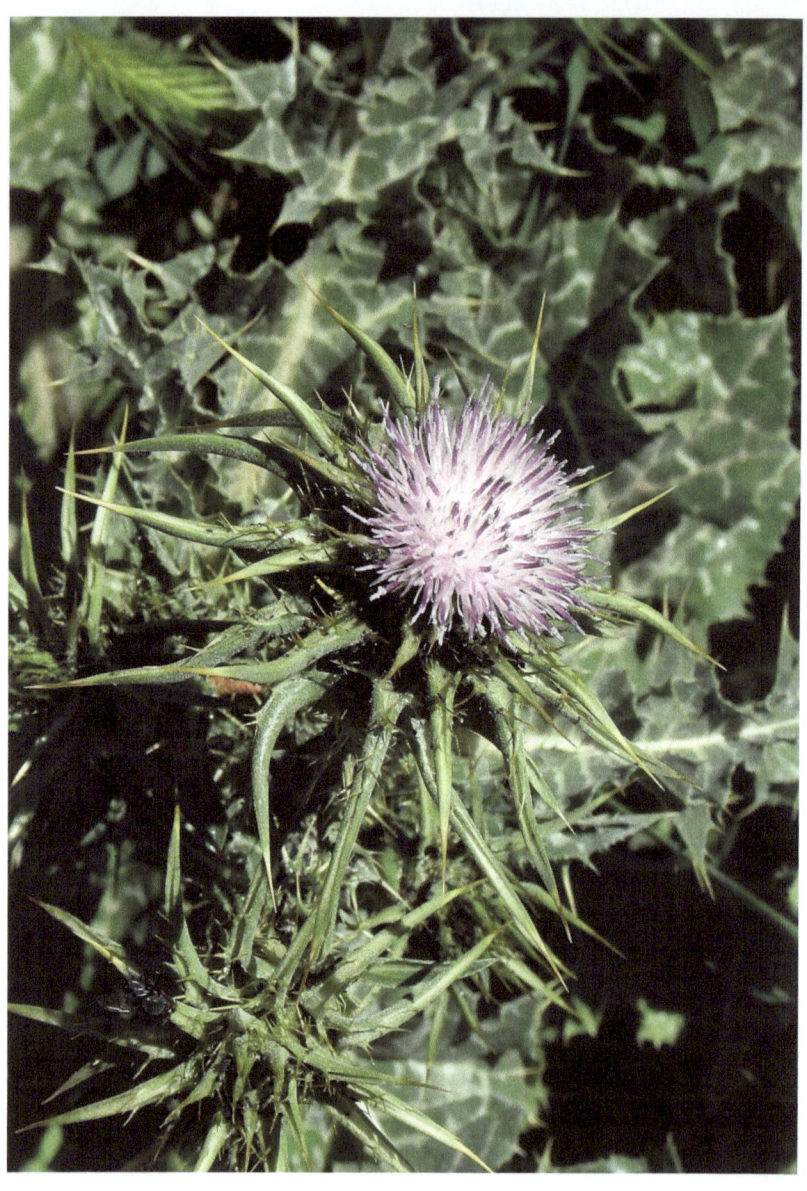

20

Milk Thistle

Description

Milk Thistles are so called because they have leaves with bands that have splashes of white color on them. The leaves are large with lobes and are waxy with thorns. The plants may be annual or biennial. The stems are tall but spineless. It produces single flowers that are pink to purple in color and shaped like a disc.

Health benefits

Milk Thistle has been used for hundreds of years as a liver tonic. It can help protect the liver and help it function well. It has been used in the case of liver diseases such as hepatitis and cirrhosis and has also been used to treat people who have ingested poisonous fungi such as the death cap mushroom. It is also thought to have anti cancer properties as well as being useful in the protection of the liver while people are undergoing chemotherapy for cancer. Milk thistle has also been used as a cure for hangovers after drinking too much alcohol.

How to use

Almost all parts of the Milk Thistle plant can be eaten and it was very popular as a food in the 1700's. The roots can be eaten raw or cooked. This can be done by boiling and then adding butter or part boiling and then roasting. The young Milk Thistle shoots can be cut in the spring and then also cooked and eaten with butter. The spines that make up the thistle flower can be eaten in a similar way to that in which artichokes are used. The older stems are bitter and have to be prepared by peeling and then soaking in water over night to get rid of the bitter taste before being stewed. The leaves can also be eaten in a similar way to spinach but the thorns have to be removed first. They can also be added to salads

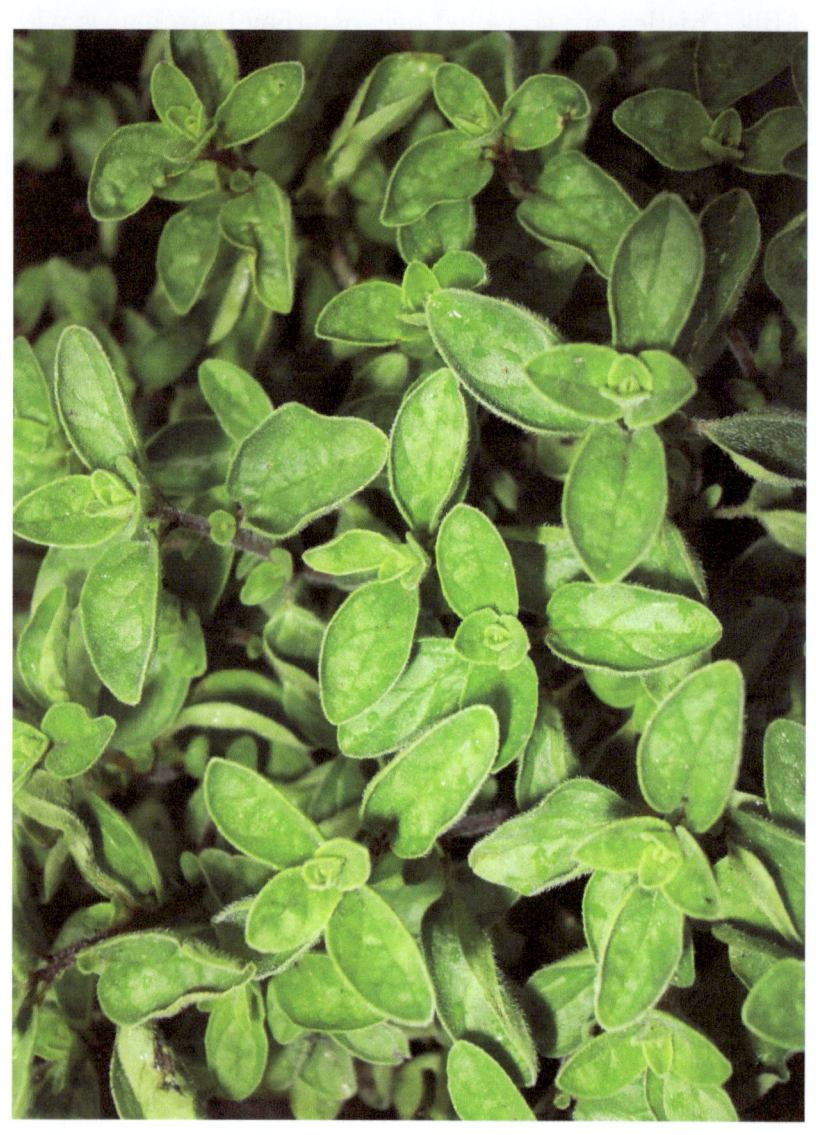

Oregano

Description

Oregano is related to Marjoram and is also referred to as wild Marjoram. It is a perennial herb and can grow to around 20 inches in height. It originates from Mediterranean regions. The leaves are grayish green and oval in shape. It produces small pink or white flowers. It has a particular warm and aromatic flavor which is slightly bitter to the taste.

Health benefits

Oregano contains a number of health promoting essential oils including thymol and carvacrol. These can help with indigestion and flatulence. Thymol also has antiseptic properties and acts as an antimicrobial. Oregano is rich in antioxidants such as vitamin A, carotenes and lutein.

This herb helps to promote digestive enzyme secretions which improve digestion. It is also a very good source of minerals including potassium, calcium and manganese. Fresh leaves of this herb contain vitamin C and as a result it has been proposed that it is also good as a treatment for the common cold.

How to use

Oregano is best added to meals late on in food preparation in order to maintain its characteristic flavor and aroma. It has been used in a variety of Mediterranean and Mexican dishes for thousands of years. Pizzas, chicken, meat and fish dishes all benefit from the addition of Oregano. It can also be used in sauces, soups omelets and as a flavoring when pickling. The raw fresh leaves can be added to green salads and even fruit salads.

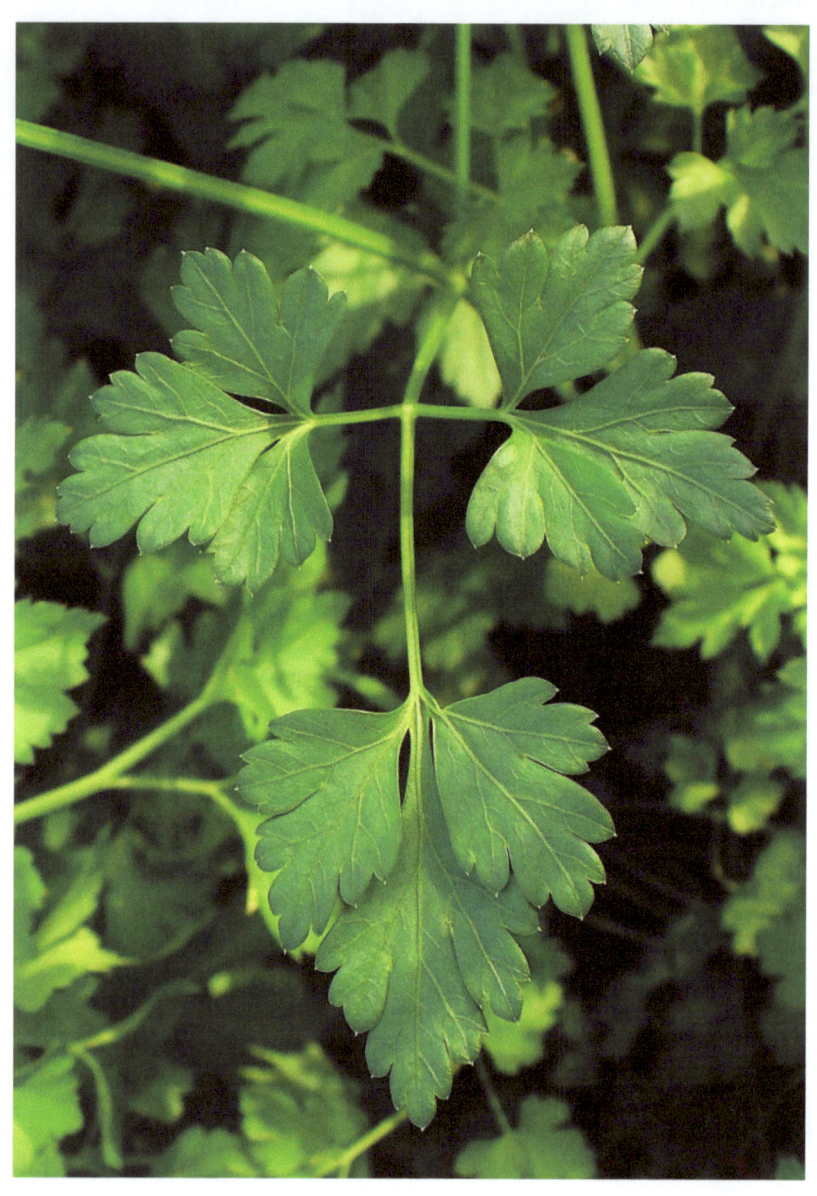

Parsley

Description

Parsley has different leaf shapes. Curly and flat leaf are popular versions. This is a biennial herb that forms a little plant with dark green leaves. The flat leaf version looks quite like coriander. It has a mild taste unlike coriander but it has a strong aroma. It originated in the Mediterranean areas.

Health benefits

Parsley has important disease preventing qualities. It contains some quality antioxidants as well. These help to deal with poisonous free radicals that build up in the body causing aging and diseases like cancer. Parsley can also help to control cholesterol levels in the blood. Parsley is also rather good at preventing constipation. It contains a number of essential oils and in particular eugenol which acts as an antiseptic in the mouth helping to deal with gum disease and teeth problems. Eugenol may also help to reduce blood sugar levels.

Parsley is rich in minerals and in particular it is high in potassium. This helps balance the other salts in the body and helps to make red blood cells.

The fresh herb contains the vitamins such as A, B complex, C, and E. It is the richest herb source for vitamin K. This vitamin helps bones to grow and repair as well as helping with Alzheimer's disease by limiting damage to nerve cells in the brain

How to use

Parsley is often chopped and used as a garnish for other dishes. It can also be a good addition to a green salad. Parsley is used a lot in Mediterranean cuisine and is often used with meat, chicken, fish and vegetables.

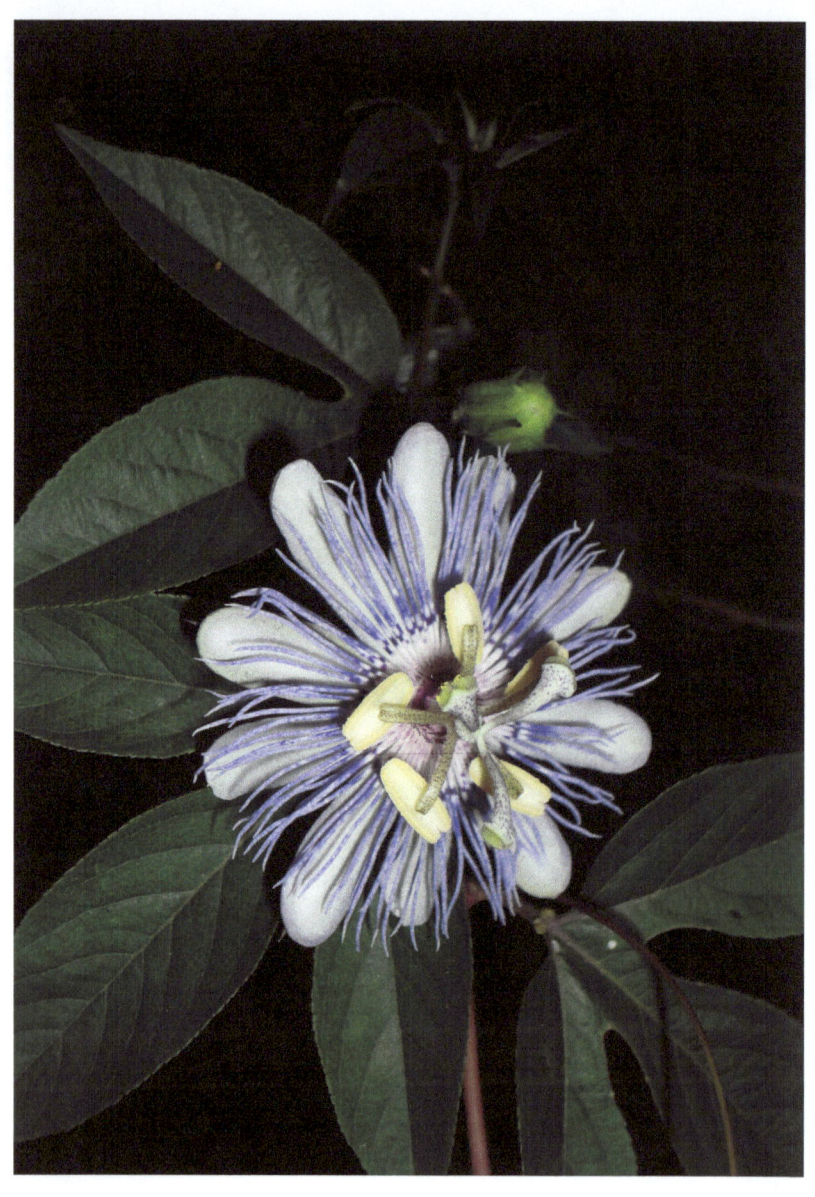

Passion Flower

Description

There are a lot of different varieties of passion flower. They occur in the Americas. It is a quick growing type of vine. The most common variety is called Maypop and is one of very few that can survive in colder locations than the tropics. The flowers themselves are so called because they were thought to be like the nails used when Christ was on the cross. Most varieties produce fruits that are round or long and may be between 2 and 8 inches long. Some varieties are cultivated purely for their fruit.

Health benefits

Passion flower was originally used by the indigenous populations of America but was later taken on by the European settlers. Tea can be made from the fresh or dried leaves. This can be used to help with insomnia and hysteria due to its calming nature. It also has pain relieving properties. Some varieties of passion flower have anti depressant properties as well.

How to use

The fruit of the passion flower is delicious and the plant has often been cultivated for the fruit alone. The leaves and roots can be made into a tea.

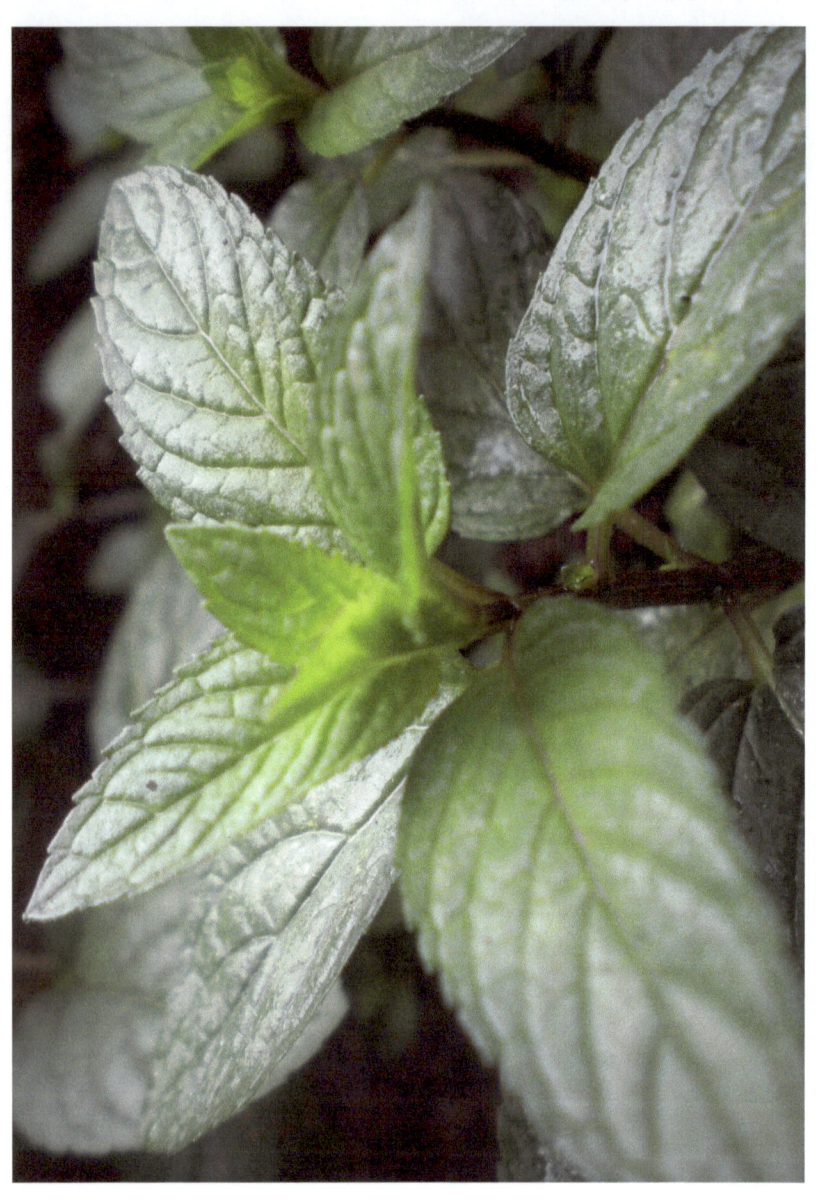

Peppermint

Description

Peppermint originated in Europe but is now grown all over the world. The dark green leaves are lance shaped and have serrated edges. It produces purple flowers. It doesn't produce seeds so it spreads by using its underground root system.

Health benefits

Peppermint produces a large number of essential oils but the main one is menthol. Due to the effect of menthol on nerve receptors in the mouth, skin and throat it causes a natural cooling reaction when it is eaten, breathed in or put on the skin. Menthol also acts as a painkiller and anti irritant. Peppermint tends to relax the walls of the digestive system and as a result people have found it helpful with irritable bowel syndrome and other conditions of the colon.

Peppermint is a good source of minerals such as potassium, calcium and iron. It also contains high levels of antioxidant vitamins such as vitamin A, C and E. The leaves are also rich in B complex vitamins such as folates. It is also a good source of vitamin K.

How to use

Peppermint can be used for cold and flu relief due to the cooling effect of the menthol. The leaves maybe eaten or steeped in hot water and the vapors breathed in. When used as a mouth wash it can help to deal with bad breath.

The Fresh herb should be used in food and drink preparation just before being consumed in order to keep its aromatic flavor and aroma at its best. You can make herbal teas from the fresh or dried leaves. It can be used as a garnish or on salads or as an ingredient in soups and sauces.

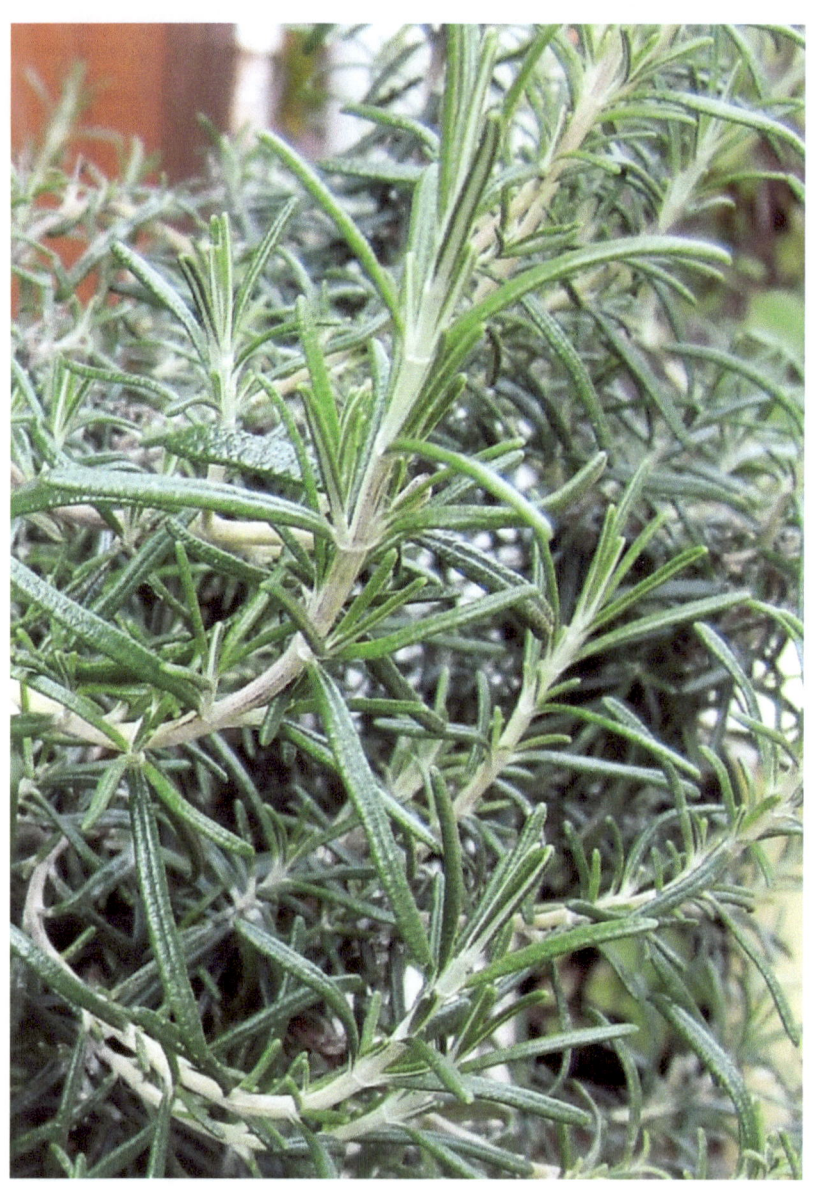

Rosemary

Description

Rosemary is a popular garden herb. It is easy to grow and being a perennial evergreen it is always there to use. It originated in the Mediterranean region. It has a woody stem and attached to this are hairy shoots to which are fixed long narrow leaves that are about one inch long, with a strong aromatic aroma. In summer it produces lots of small purple flowers.

Health benefits

Rosemary contains plant substances which have health enhancing qualities. Leaves and flower tops have rosmarinic acid and a number of essential oils within them that have health benefits. These include anti irritant and anti inflammatory properties.

Rosemary contains high levels of vitamin B complex compounds especially folates. There are also large amounts of Vitamin A which has antioxidant anti aging properties. Even a few leaves a day can provide the recommended daily amount of this vitamin. The fresh leaves contain lots of Vitamin C.

Fresh and dried Rosemary provides lots of mineral content: especially potassium, calcium, iron and manganese. It is a good source of iron which is good for making red blood cells and preventing anemia.

How to use

Rosemary should be added towards the end of cooking to prevent loss of flavor and aroma. It is popular in Mediterranean cuisine where it is used in salads, soups with meat and vegetable dishes. It goes well with tomatoes, potatoes, aubergine and courgettes. A tea can be made to help with colds, headache and depression.

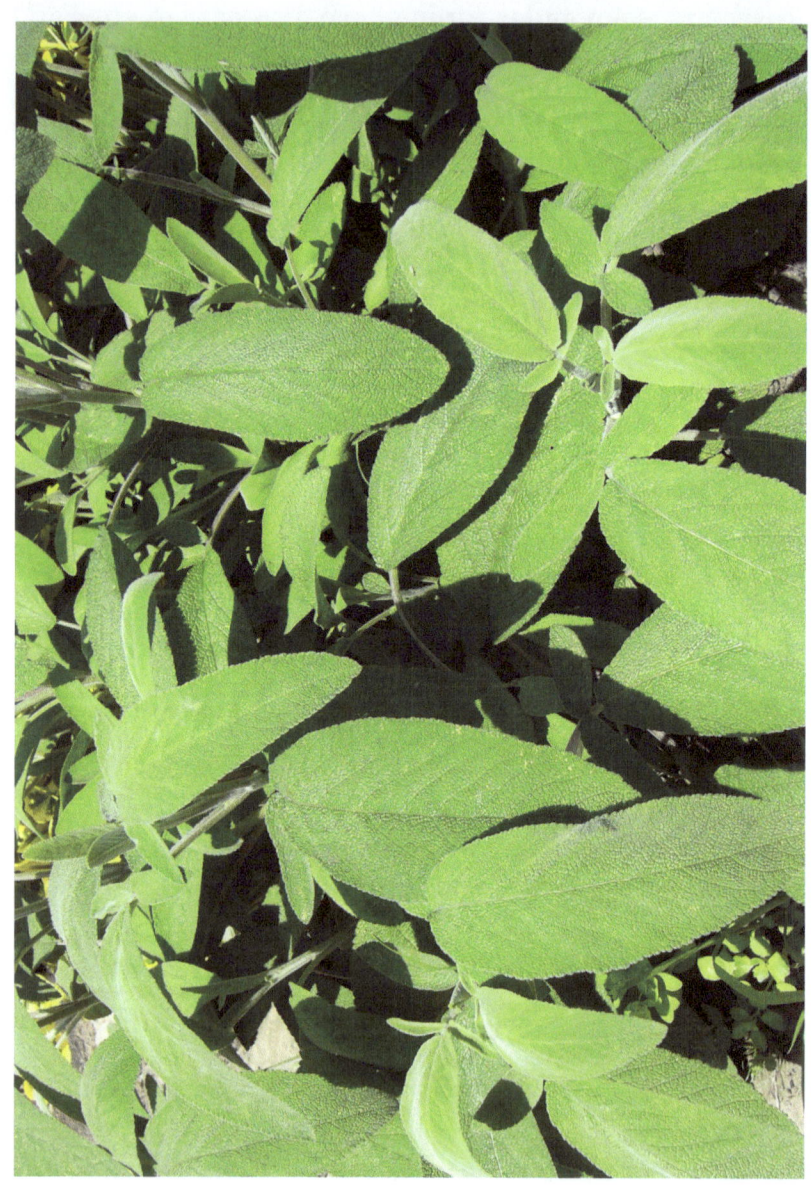

32

Sage

Description

Sage has been in use since the times of the Roman Empire. It is a perennial herb which is found as a shrub in the Mediterranean and Eastern Europe. Its branching woody stems can grow as high as 75 cm. The leaves are aromatic and greenish grey in color. They have fine hairs growing on both sides of the leaves. It produces bunches of blue to violet colored flowers in the summer months.

Health benefits

Sage contains the essential oil Thujone and many other compounds such as cineol, tannic acid and nicotinic acids. These all combine to give it anti irritant, anti inflammatory and antiseptic qualities. Thujone tends to increase concentration and quickens the senses. Tea made from sage is said top help you think as well as helping with depression.

It is rich in vitamins including B complex and is a good source of Vitamin C. It also contains high levels of the minerals potassium, zinc, calcium and iron.

The oil from sage when rubbed onto affected areas is good at soothing pain in muscles, stiffness, rheumatism and neuralgia. When used as a massage oil it can help with headaches, nervousness and anxiety.

How to use

Sage is a sharply flavored herb and is used a lot in Italian, Greek and Eastern European cooking. It is a common ingredient for stuffing for such foods as sausage, fish and poultry. It can also be used with beans and many other vegetable recipes. Use as a garnish in salads and with roast pork.

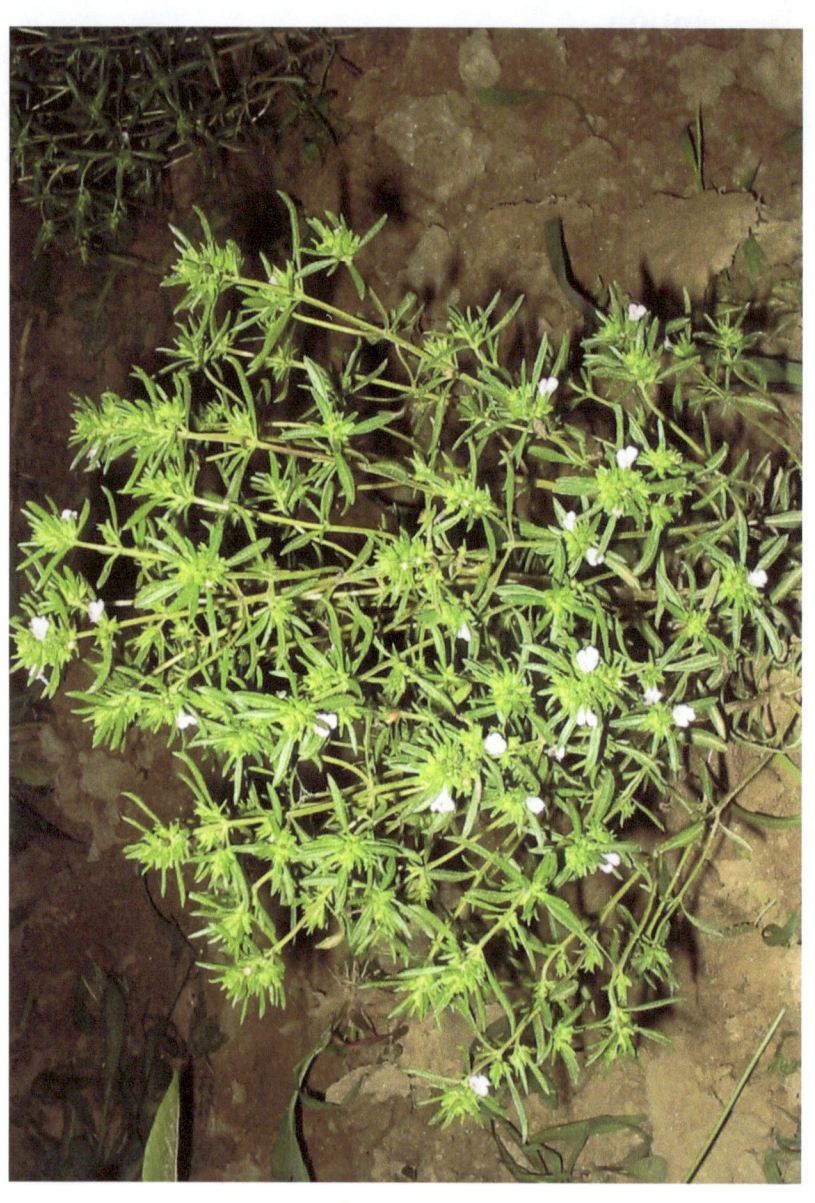

34

Savory

Description

Summer Savory is a weakly aromatic and nice herb which is used a lot in American and Eastern European cooking. In good sunlight it can grow to about 2 feet in height. It has dark green leaves with quite a smooth texture. It produces little flowers that are purple in color. Winter savory is similar, but more aromatic in taste and the stems are woodier in structure.

Health benefits

Savory has many good essential oils which have been found to act against bacteria and fungi. A water infusion can be used for gargling to help with sore throats and bronchitis type conditions. The leaves and herbal shoots can help with flatulence, digestion, coughs and joint pains.

Thymol and Carvacrol are the active ingredients that have the most anti microbial activity. Carvacrol gives a nice tangy and aromatic flavor to any food that it has been used in.

It is rich in vitamins such as B complex, A and C. It contains vitamin B6 which can help with dealing with stress due to its actions on the nervous system.

How to use

Savory leaves used in cooking give a weak peppery and tangy flavor. It tastes a little like marjoram. It should be used towards the end of cooking in order to preserve its flavor. The fresh leaves can be used as garnish for salads. A herbal tea can be made from Savory leaves and this has proved to be a popular health drink. It can be used in the making of soups and sauces. With other herbs and spices, it can be used to marinate fish, chicken and meat dishes.

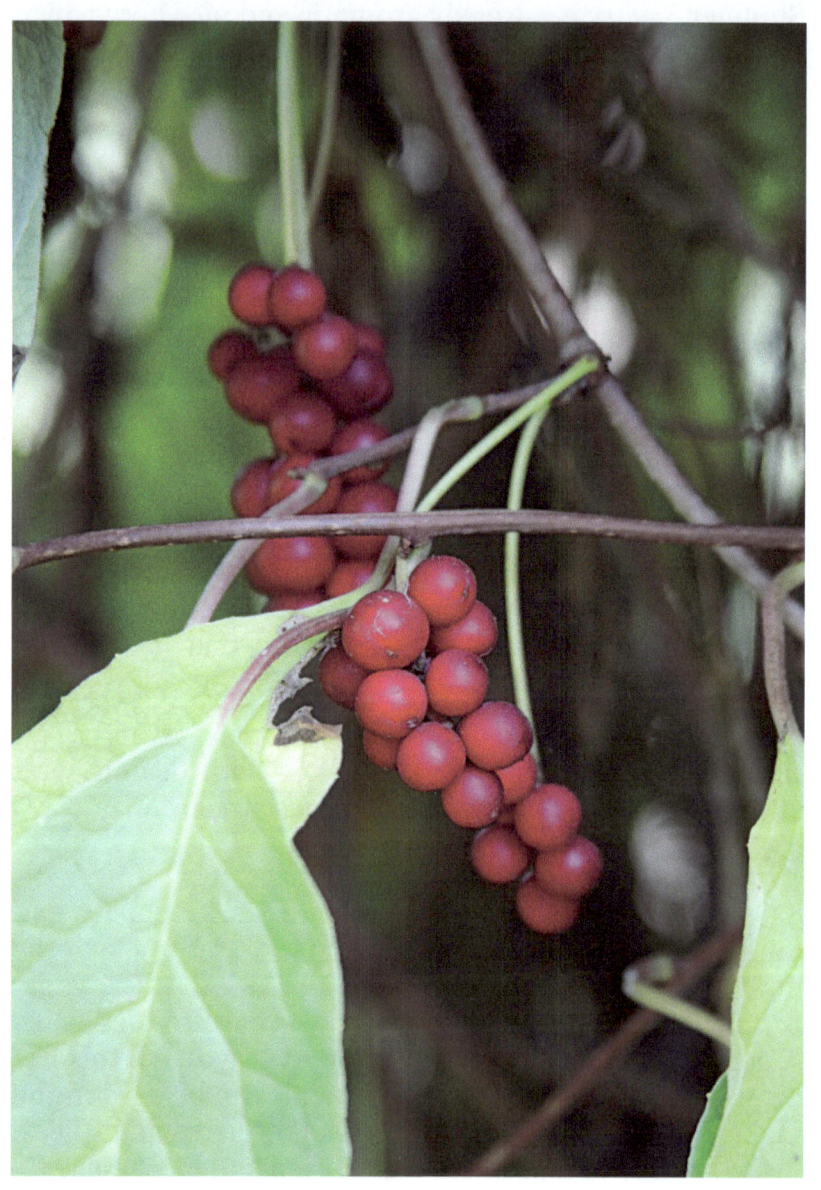

Schizandra

Description

Schizandra produces red berries that are said to have the five flavors in one. The plant producing the berries is natives to China and Eastern Russia. It is a woody vine that loses its leaves in winter time. It can be grown in similar regions in the US. In Russia the berries are harvested in huge numbers and used to produce juices, wines and sweets.

Health benefits

Schizandra has been widely used in Chinese medicine for thousands of years. It can be used to increase a person's ability to work and as an agent to deal with a number of harmful factors such as frostbite, heavy metal poisoning, heat shock and sunburn.

The Russians use it to improve night vision and to put off feelings of hunger.

The Japanese use it for treating colds and sea sickness.

The Chinese use it in the treatment of diarrhea and calming of the spirit.

Schizandra improves the functioning of the liver and can help with blood sugar levels and blood pressure.

How to use

Schizandra is usually used in the dry form where the berries are boiled in water to make a tea. You can buy the dried fruit from most health shops and online.

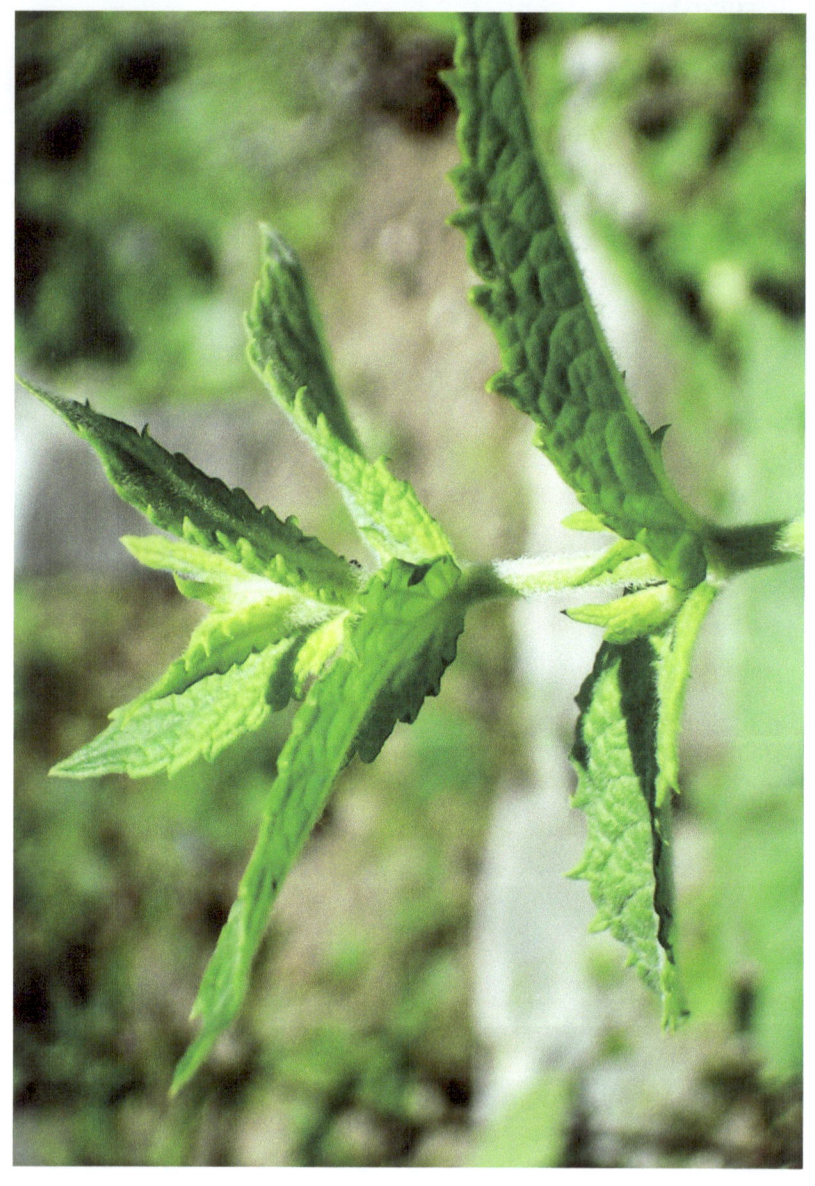

Spearmint

Description

Spearmint is also known as garden mint. It originates from the Mediterranean region where it grows as a perennial. The leaves are mainly used and are large, dark green and oval in shape. Spearmint plants can grow to about 75cm in height. They are serrated and have ends that are pointed. Flowers are produced in summer and are mauve in color.

Health benefits

Spearmint decoction can be used to treat headaches, tiredness and stress. Spearmint can also be used to combat digestive problems such as flatulence, feeling sick and hiccups because of the way that it relaxes the muscles of the digestive tract. The essential oil menthol in the herb can help with irritations and also aches and pains. Applying it to the skin can help with itching and dermatitis.

How to use

Spearmint is well known for the specific aroma that it adds to the foods in which it is included. Spearmint can be boiled in water to extract the essential ingredients as a decoction. Spearmint oil can be used during massage to relieve stress and aches. Chopped fresh leaves can be added to salads and as a garnish for other dishes. Mint sauce can be made either using yoghurt or vinegar as the base. It can be used as a flavoring for such things as ice cream and other sweet dishes. Spearmint leaf tea is a popular health drink. During cooking spearmint is normally added towards the end of food preparation and in small amounts.

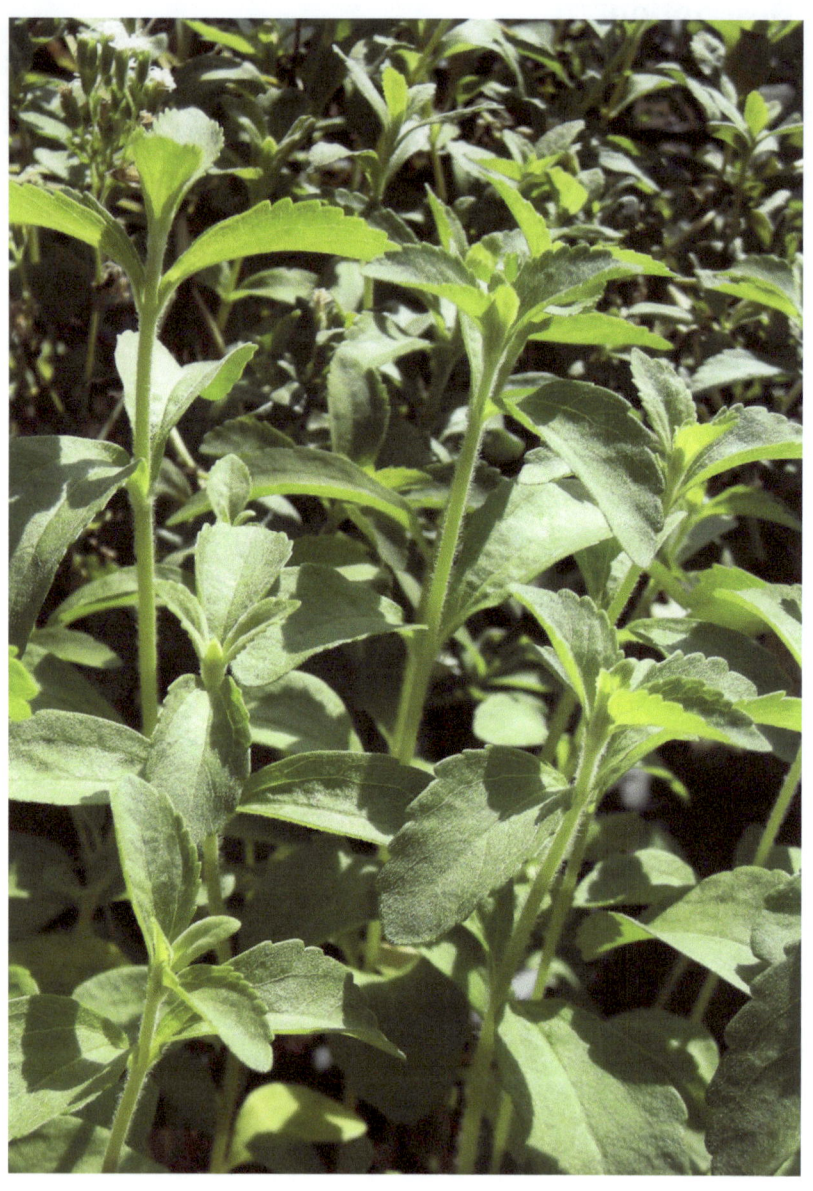

Stevia

Description

Stevia is a small herb from South America that has sweet leaves. It has been used by the natives of Paraguay for centuries. It grows to around a metre in height and has thin branched stems. It has dark green leaves where the majority of the sweet taste is located. It is now grown throughout the world where local conditions are similar to Paraguay.

Health benefits

Stevia has been used traditionally to treat conditions such as wounds, inflammation and swelling in the limbs. It can be used as a way of losing weight as well as to treat depression.

The main use is as a sweetener because it is low in calories but has roughly 40 times the sweetness power of table sugar.

Some sterols in Stevia are thought to help in the fight against cancer.

Chlorogenic acid within the herb can help to control blood sugar levels.

Some glycoside compounds in Stevia can help to widen blood vessels and in so doing can help to reduce blood pressure.

In Brazil it is widely used to treat such conditions as high blood pressure, diabetes and stress.

How to use

Fresh Stevia leaves can be used in drinks directly as a sweetener but it is more usual to use extracts of the leaf.

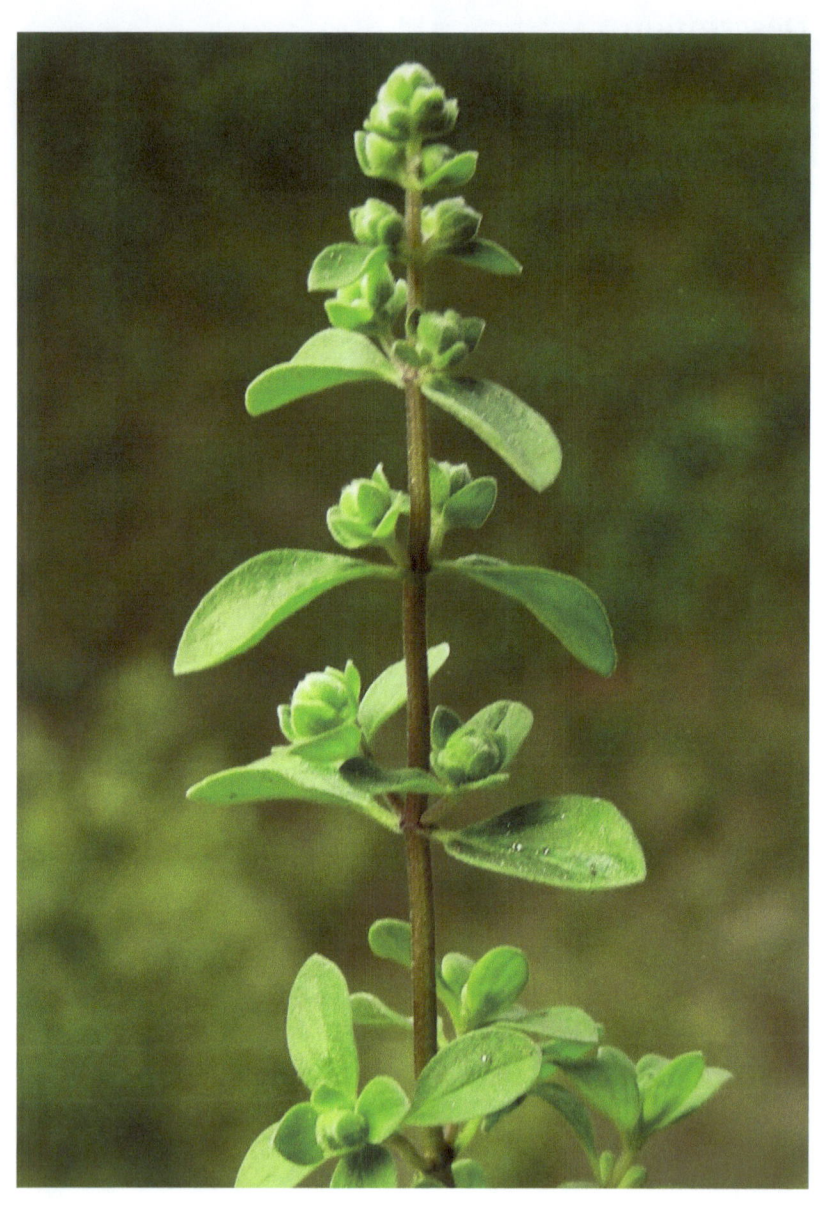

Sweet Marjoram

Description

Marjoram is a popular herb in the Mediterranean region and has been used for both food dishes and health issues. It has been used in this way since olden times. It has a fine sweet taste and is slightly spicy. It originally came from Turkey but is now grown throughout the Mediterranean region. It is a small and woody shrub and grows to about 80cm in height. The dark green oval shaped leaves are supported on a hairy stem. It produces little white and pink flowers.

Health benefits

Marjoram has a number of essential oils that have health benefits. The main ones are terpenes, linalool and carvocrol. These oils have anti inflammatory and anti microbial properties. Marjoram can be used to treat pain in the muscles, rheumatism and flatulence.

It contains the substance eugenol which can be used to treat arthritis and certain bowel conditions due to its inflammatory properties.

It can be used to help reduce pains during menstruation.

A tea can be made to help with feelings of sickness and flatulence.

How to use

Marjoram can be used in salads, stews, soups and marinades where it adds extra flavor. It can also be used in vegetable and egg recipes. It gives a nice aromatic flavor to cauliflower, spinach, tomatoes, peas, beans, carrots and potatoes. You can mix it with a lot of other different herbs. It is often added to sausages, pizza and poultry stuffing.

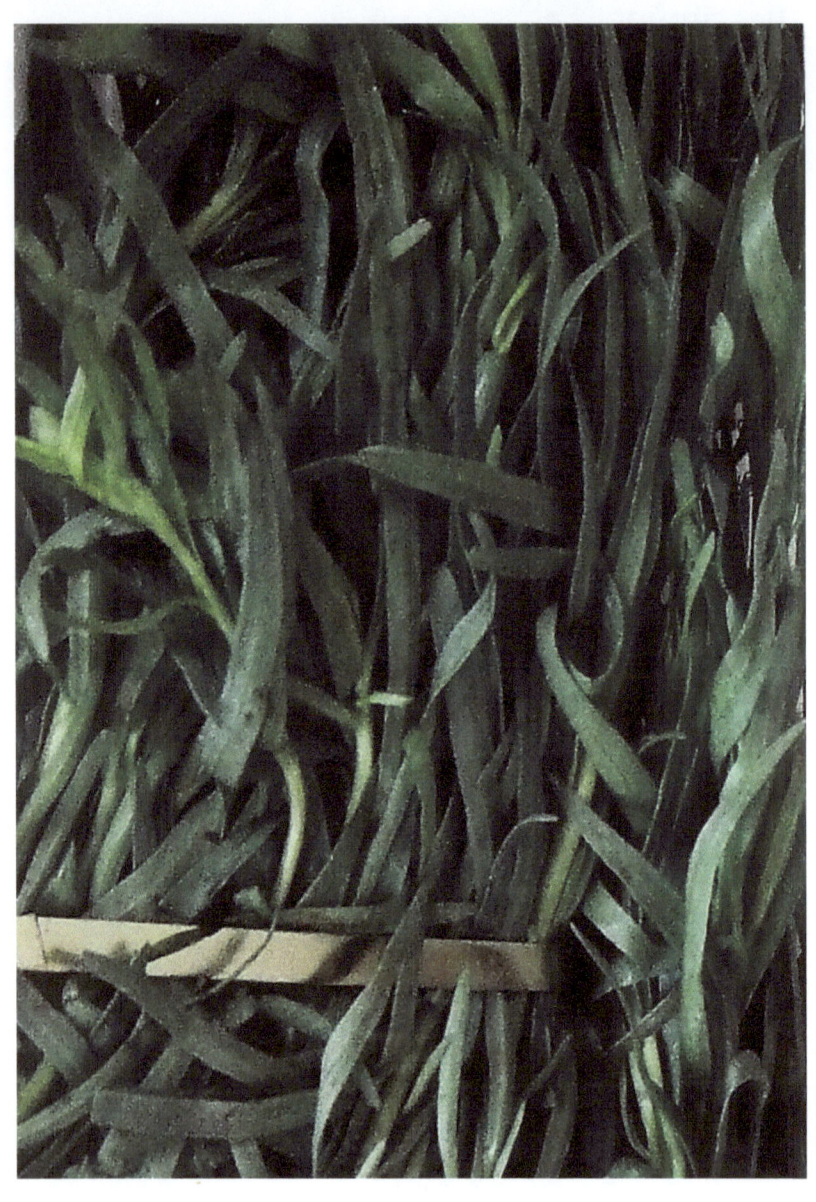

Tarragon

Description

Tarragon is a popular herb in the Mediterranean region. It is thought to have originally come from Siberia where it still exists but as an inferior version compared to that currently grown in the Mediterranean. It is found as a small perennial shrub up to 1 metre in height. It has branching stems. The leaves have pointed ends and are dark green with a smooth surface texture.

Health benefits

Tarragon is rich in health giving nutrients such as antioxidants which can help fight disease and maintain health.

The main active ingredient in this herb is the essential oil called estragole.

Tarragon can be used to stimulate appetite and may even be of help in preventing anorexic symptoms. Poly phenolic compounds in this herb may help to reduce blood sugar levels.

Extracts of Tarragon have been shown to prevent blood cells sticking together as clots and then sticking to blood vessel walls. This has led to its use in preventing strokes and heart disease.

It has a wide range of vitamins and minerals and is a good source of vitamin C, calcium, manganese and iron.

How to use

Tarragon tea may be used to help with problems sleeping.

Fresh Tarragon leaves can be used as an ingredient in green salads. It can be used in marinades for fish, poultry and lamb dishes.

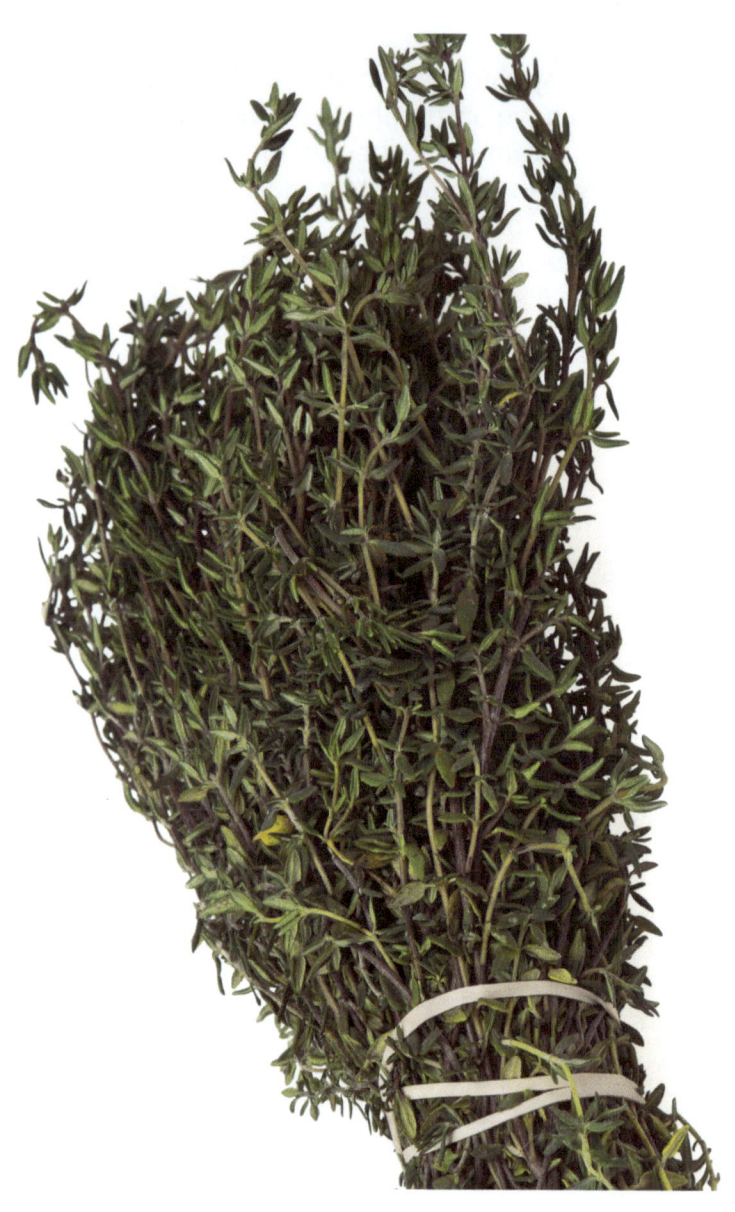

46

Thyme

Description

Thyme contains lots of health giving plant substances including vitamins and minerals which are important for maintaining a healthy body. Thyme originally came from Southern Europe. It grows as a perennial herb. It has a thick main woody base and the stems are square in shape. It can grow up to 25 cm in height and has small green leaves that are not as dark underneath. White or lilac flowers are produced in the summer months.

Health benefits

Thyme contains the essential oil thymol which has anti microbial properties.

It has a number of antioxidants including lutein and thymonin which can help prevent ageing in the cells of the body

Thyme has high levels of essential minerals such as potassium, manganese, iron and calcium. It is also a good source of the vitamins B, A, C, E and K.

It can be used as a gargle to help with colds, coughs and sore throats.

How to use

Thyme can be made into a refreshing tea which is a popular health drink in many parts of the world.

You can use Thyme when making soups and sauces. It can be used as part of marinades used on poultry, fish and meat. It can also be added as an ingredient for stuffing used with chicken and fish.

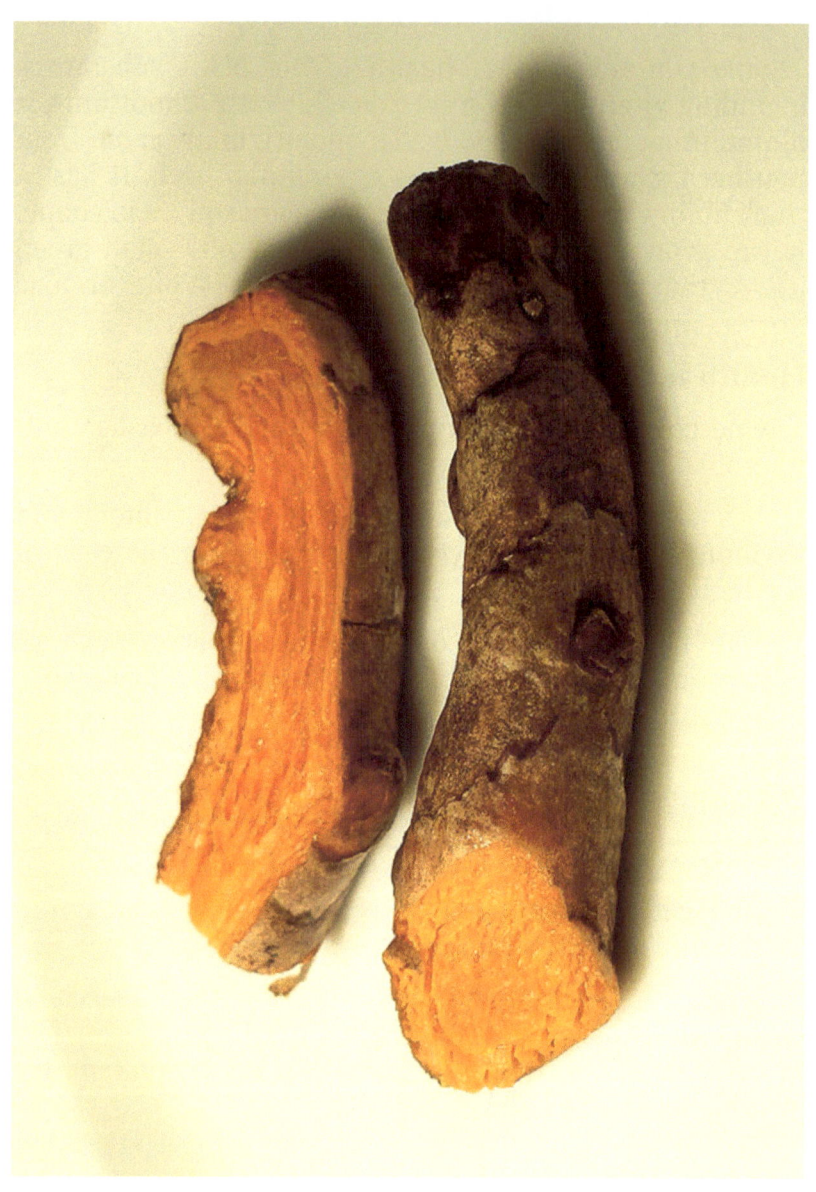

Turmeric

Description

Turmeric roots and leaves have been used in medicine and cooking for centuries. Originally from the Himalayan mountains it is now cultivated in many parts of the world. Turmeric can grow up to a metre in height and has aromatic leaves. The roots have a dark brown skin which surrounds an orange colored flesh. Both leaves and roots have the same weakly pepper and bitter, warm taste. The aroma given off is nice and sweet which is a bit like a mixture of orange and ginger.

Health benefits

Turmeric root has traditionally used for its anti inflammatory and pain killer properties. It can also combat flatulence and has anti microbial qualities.

Curcumin is the name given to the orange pigment of Turmeric and this may have properties to help deal with certain cancers. It is recommended by some doctors as part of an anti cancer diet, which may be taken to prevent cancers or after cancer treatments in hospital. Curcumin may also be of use treating inflammation and arthritis.

Turmeric is rich in vitamins and contains a wide spectrum of minerals. Fresh Turmeric root is a good source of vitamin C.

Turmeric contains health giving essential oils such as termerone and curlone.

How to use

Turmeric can be used in the marinating of fish, meat, chicken and shell fish. It is used in India in curry dishes. It can be used in the making of soups and dressings for salads. In some parts of the world Turmeric tea is a popular drink.

About The Author

Ellen Vincent has written a number of other books that you may well be interested in. They are all about healthy living and the use of natural products to enhance our lives. These books have been written from the personal experience of using the products and seeing how good that they can be for us. Go to the web pages listed for further information on each book. The books are available as paperbacks and in the Kindle format.

Apple Cider Vinegar for Natural Health

http://www.amazon.com/Apple-Cider-Vinegar-Natural-Health/dp/1475220707/

Green Smoothie Recipes

www.amazon.com/Green-Smoothie-Recipes-ingredients-ingredient/dp/1480124117/

Green Smoothie: Diet, Detox and Recipes

http://www.amazon.com/Green-Smoothie-Diet-Detox-Recipes/dp/1475179731/

Coconut Oil

http://www.amazon.com/Coconut-Oil-including-coconut-benefits/dp/1481261835/

www.ingramcontent.com/pod-product-compliance
Lightning Source LLC
Chambersburg PA
CBHW050831290526
45792CB00001B/354